AYURVEDA FOR ORAL HEALTH

DR. AMIT A. PATIL

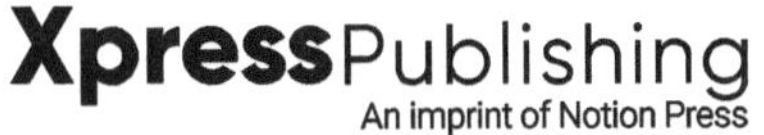

XpressPublishing
An imprint of Notion Press

Old No. 38, New No. 6
McNichols Road, Chetpet
Chennai - 600 031

First Published by Notion Press 2020
Copyright © Dr. Amit A. Patil 2020
All Rights Reserved.

ISBN 978-1-64869-378-6

Dedicated

To My Grandmother Late Smt Indumati Raghunath Patil

Contents

Preface

Ayurveda is a science of life which deals with preventive aspect for human being since five thousand years. Ayurveda mentioned that who follows rules of health prevention as given in samhita texts, lives for full span of life with healthy and good quality of life.

It is observed that oral health problems in a society remarkably increased now a day. Also modern health system is very costly. Oral health is window of all over health. Healthy mouth can help to ward of medical disorders. Therefore this book is filled with knowledge for leading a healthy oral cavity through traditional Ayurveda point of view. All topics are listed separately so that it becomes easier to understand. All the things mention in this book are helpful to common people and Ayurveda students who will research in field oral health.

Also I requested to common people to follow some ayurvedic traditional methods in daily routine for maintaining healthy oral cavity. I am waiting for your suggestions.

DR AMIT ASHOK PATIL

Acknowledgements

I have a great pleasure while keeping this book in front of reputed personalities in the society. I take this opportunity as a deep sense of gratitude to those people and institution that helped me during this publication of book.

I am very much thankful to my colleague **Dr.Santosh Swami (HOD, Department of Kayachikitsa)** for their encouragement and moral support. I am grateful to **Dr.Vidula Patil** my wife and co-auther of this book for her valuable support. Also I am very much thankful to my friends **Dr Vipul Patil, Dr Rakesh Shukla,Dr Dhananjay Patil, Dr Archana**for their valuable help and support.

Lastly and most importantly I offer my regards to **My Father Ashok Patil, My Mother Mrs. Dr Maya Patil, My Brother Dentist Dr Abhay Patil,** family relatives, each and every person directly or indirectly involved in this work. Without whose support and blessings this book would have not seen the light of day.

DR AMIT

ASHOK PATIL

HOD AND

ASSOCIATE PROFESSOR

DEPATMENT OF

SWASTHAVRITTA EVAM YOGA

MES AYURVED

MAHAVIDYALAYA,GHANEKHUNT- LOTE

(MAHARASHTRA)

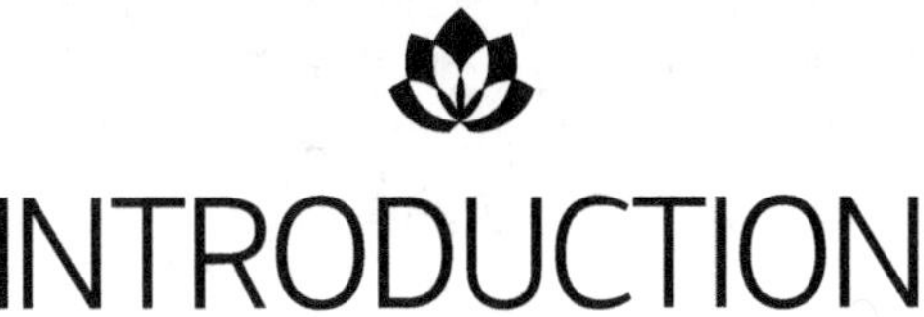

CHAPTER ONE

INTRODUCTION

Health and health problems are challenging issues in modern lifestyle. Civilization has raised major lifestyle disorders through the use of synthetic contents in daily care products in spite of natural products. Use of natural things in daily regimen is important for good health and for that Ayurveda is solution!

The decisive aim of any medical science is for attainment of level of health, which enables every individual to lead socially and economically productive life. In this regard Ayurveda stands first, as it is the science of life, which primarily aims at preservation of positive health.

Oral diseases are one of the most important problems in public health. Oral health also reflects the overall physical and mental health. The Global Burden of Disease Study 2016 estimated that oral diseases affected half of the world's population.

WHO defines oral health as "a state of being free from chronic mouth and facial pain, oral and throat cancer, oral infection and sores, periodontal (gum) disease, tooth decay, tooth loss, and other diseases and disorders that limit an individual's capacity in biting, chewing, smiling, speaking, and psychosocial well being."

This concept of oral health is best achieved through Ayurveda. Ayurveda is conventional source for oral health. This traditional system of medicine not only recommends treatments with specific herbs and minerals to cure various oral diseases but also recommends some daily therapeutic procedures for the prevention and maintenance of oral health along with safety and effectiveness. Recently, there is renewed interest in use of various Ayurveda drugs and therapeutic procedures for oral and dental health. Ayurveda recommends and insist on the use of herbal brushes. Chewing sticks, *Gandusha, Kawala* (swish), *Jivhalekhana* (Tongue cleaning) are traditional methods have been widely used in the India since past.

These methods are cost effective and closer to the community. No specialist required to follow the procedures as these can be adopted easily in routine with thorough knowledge. With this book one is able to adopt these procedures in routine with more scientific way. Also World Health Organization has initiated the awareness regarding the oral health and use of Ayurveda for oral health. According to World health Organization (WHO) 75% of the world's population uses herbs for basic health care needs. WHO has recommended for the incorporation of the traditional systems of medicine like Ayurveda into the primary health care system, for those communities where it is accepted. All the Ayurveda medicines and local remedies are easily available in the rural areas where socioeconomic condition of the people is not good enough to buy costly toothpaste or curative medicines. Ayurveda must be reinterpreted in the light of our new knowledge and it must be incorporated in modern medicine along with other forms of traditional medicine. For all these achievements this book is source of light for common peoples.

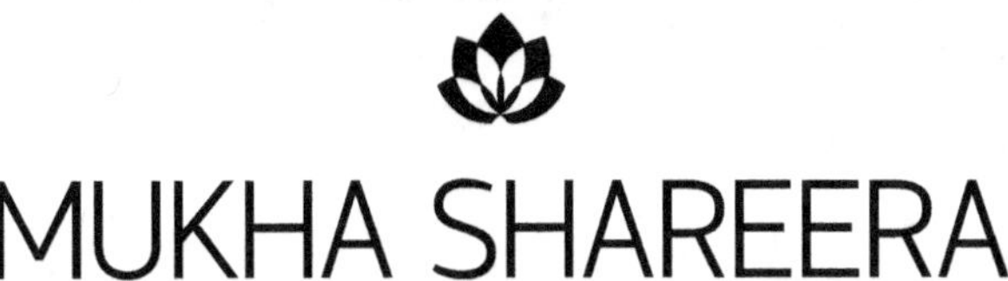

CHAPTER TWO

MUKHA SHAREERA

The meaning, synonym and description of Ayurvedic terms are described below.

Nirukti and *paryaya* of mukha

"Khanyate bhakshate anena iti mukham"

It means the part that helps in eating.

Synonyms:

1. *Vadanam.*
2. *Vaktram.*
3. *Tundam.*
4. *Aasyam.*
5. *Ananam.*
6. *Lapanam.*

Vadanam – 'Vadanti iti vadanam' i.e. Which helps in speaking.

Vaktram – 'Uchchate anena iti vaktram'

Means part that helps in speaking.

Tundam – *Tudyate himsate iti tundam.*

Which helps in breaking.

shapane **Asyam**– *Asu kor aasyam mukha kuharam.*

Which helps in eating.

Ananam – *Aniti shwasate anena iti.*

Which helps in breathing.

Lapanam – That helps in speaking.

From the above explanations, it is clear that mukha is the part of body, which helps in eating, speaking and breathing; hence we consider it as the oral cavity.

Garbha shareera—during garbha vriddhi mukha is formed in fifth month.

Pramana shareera---Pramana of mukha is four or five angula·

Mukha Pratyangas

Mukha includes the fallowing structures.

1. Oshta - lips
2. Dantamoola – gums
3. Danta- teeth
4. Jiwha – tongue
5. Talu- soft and hard palate
6. Gala- oropharynx
7. Kapola - cheeks

According to Yogratnakar and Sushrut Samhita, Mukha (oral cavity) consists of lips, gums, teeth, tongue, palate and throat.Mukha is that organ of the body, which meant, for ingestion of food. Taste recognized by tongue and accordingly saliva secretion occurs. Food is masticated by teeth, are mixed with saliva and swallowing of food occurs with the help of tongue and hard palate.

OSHTHA (LIPS) :

Lips are the fleshy folds, which close the mouth cavity. Lips are the Matruj organs.

SIGNS OF SWASTHA (HEALTHY) LIPS:

Lips length should be 4 Anguli. Lips should not be so thick and should not be so thin. Mouth should be open after joining both the lips. Normal lips colour should be like riped bimba fruit. The lip of the Raktasar man has delicate, unctuous and dark red coloued. A lip of the Medasar man has unctuous.

DANTA (TEETH)

Danta known as "ruchaka-asthi" and is variety of bony tissue. The word "ruchaka" means which imparts taste & "asthi" means bone. Thus, ruchaka-asthi means bones associated with function of imparting taste. Teeth are Pitruj organs & parts of prithvi (Earth) mahabhuta are more in them.There are 32 permanent teeth and 24 primary deciduous teeth. The central incisors, lateral incisors, the canines and molars called as Rajadanta, Vasta and Danshtra and 6 of Hanavya respectively. There are 2 each of Rajadanta, Vasta and 6 of Hanavya in each upper & lower jaw.

NORMAL TEETH AND GUMS:

Normal healthy teeth are strong, white dense, smooth, clean, slightly prominent, well developed , evenly placed in relation to each other. They do not decay and not affected by diseases. The gums are even, pink, smooth, strong, dense and steady.

DOSHAS PRESENT IN TEETH

Vata, Pitta and Kapha all the three doshas which are present in tooth; but since tooth is type of bone, Vata is more dominant. If Vata alleviated, tooth becomes weak & cavitiesformed. If vata is in normal condition, teeth are healthy.

DHATUS PRESENT IN DANTA

Rasa Dhatu –

Normal rasdhatu produces other dhatus in normal state.

Rakta Dhatu–

 Gums are pinkish red due to raktadhatu.

Mamsa Dhatu-

It covers root of teeth & protects gums. If gums are normal, teeth are normal. If Mansa dhatu is not normal, body gets weak and gums become inflamed. Also bleeding and pus discharge starts. It results in loosening of teeth.

Meda Dhatu –

Because of Meda Dhatu, teeth are unctuous & shining. It also protects gums & so gums tightened & hold teeth firmly. If meda Dhatu pacified, fat reduced and due to abnormal vata, teeth break and cavities & caries formed.

Asthi Dhatu-

Teeth made up of asthi. The condition of teeth is dependent on condition of asthi dhatu. If asthi dhatu is sarwan, teeth are big, strong & hard. If asthi dhatu is not normal there is gap between teeth. Teeth get cracked and pain is present. In asthivridhi, overlapping of teeth on normal teeth occurs.

Majja Dhatu-

The deepness & strength of root in gums is dependent on majja dhatu. If majja dhatu is sarwan, joint is deep & strong. Cavity filled with danta majja, which gives strength to teeth. If this danta majja is not normal, then formation of dental caries with pain and insomnia occurs.

Shukradhatu-

The teeth of shukrasara person are healthy, similar, shiny, without gaps, in one line & beautiful like pearls. If shukra dhatu is healthy, teeth eruption occurs at proper age. After falling primary teeth, permanent teeth are erupted without any trouble. In age 12 to 25 years, shukra dhatu is in fully mature stage. In this age only, wisdom tooth erupts. This shows relation of shukra dhatu and teeth.

Talu- Palate (hard palate)

"   *Tarantyanena Varna iti talu*"

That helps in pronouncing varnas

"   *Talati pratishtati pishtadikamatra talu*"

The part which encapsulates food while chewing
Synonym - Kakudam

" *Kakum dhvanirvisheshan dadati iti Kakudam*"

That which gives the voice of specificity.
In classics we get reference regarding Talu mamsa which we can consider as soft palate.

Galam (Oropharynx)

"   *Galati grasam anena galaha*"

That which helps in deglutition
Greeva

"   *Grasam girati iti griva*"

That which helps to fall i.e. that helps the food to fall in to the oesophagus
Kapolam (cheeks)

"   *Kampate iti kapolam.*"

One which shows movement
Jiwha (tongue)

" *Ledhi lihantyanaya veti jiwha* "

The one which helps for licking the food substance.

Synonym

Rasana -- Rasa asvadane

" *Rasayati va rasana* "

The one which helps in perception of taste i.e. rasavishaya grahana

Parts of Jiwha

We get scattered references of anatomical parts of jiwha in classics in various contexts they are: -

- Jiwha sevani – frenulam linguae
- Jiwha talam – under surface of tongue
- Jiwhagram – tip of tongue
- Jiwhamulam – base of tongue(posterior $1/3^{rd}$ part of tongue)

CHAPTER THREE

ANATOMY OF ORAL CAVITY

Introduction to mouth

Mouth is the only part of the alimentary canal involved in ingestion or food entry in to the body. Within the mouth food is chewed, mixed and moistened with saliva, containing enzymes that begin the process of digestion

Anatomy of Mouth

The mouth, a mucosa lined cavity is also called the oral cavity or Buccal (bucca-cheeks) cavity. It is formed by cheeks laterally, soft and hard palate superiorly. Anterior opening is oral orifice. Posteriorly it is continuous with the oropharynx.

Anatomically oral cavity is divided into two parts.

1) Vestibule of oral cavity
2) Oral cavity proper

1) Vestibule of oral cavity

It is space bounded externally by the cheeks and lips and internally by gums and teeth.

2) Oral cavity proper

It is the space that extends from the gums and teeth to the fouces (opening

between oral cavity and pharynx

Structures coming under oral cavity

1) Vestibule of oral cavity—Cheeks, Lips, Gum, Teeth
   2) Oral cavity proper-- Tongue, Soft palate, hard palate, Oro pharynx and Salivary glands

Cheeks

These are muscular structures covered externally by skin and internally by non keratinized stratified squamous epithelium. The anterior portion of the cheeks end at the lips. Cheeks are formed by buccinatars. In the walls of the cheeks fibrous tissue, vessels nerves and numerous small Buccal, mucous (salivary glands) are situated.

Cheeks help in keeping food between the teeth when we chew and play a small role in speech.

Lips

The lips (labia) are fleshy folds surrounding the opening of the mouth. They are covered externally by skin and internally by a mucous membrane. The orbicularis oris muscle forms the bulk of the fleshy lips.

Anatomically lips extend from the inferior margin of the nose to superior boundary of the chin. The reddened area where one applies the lipstick is called the red margin. This is the transitional zone where the highly keratinized skin meets the oral mucosa. There is no sweat or sebaceous glands in the red margin. So it must be moistened with saliva periodically to prevent it from dry and cracked.

The labial phrenulum is a median fold that joins the internal aspect of each lip to the gum. during chewing contraction of buccinators muscle in the cheeks and orbicularis oris muscle in lips help to keep the food between upper and lower teeth.

The labial glands situated between the mucosa and orbicularis oris are about the size of small peas and in structure resemble mucous salivary glands.

Gums (Gingivae)

The gums are composed of dense vascular fibrous tissue and are normally covered by orthokeratinized stratified squamous epithelium. They are firmly attached to the cement at the neck of the neck and to the bones of adjacent alveolar process. Gums get nerve supply from maxillary nerve via its various branches like grater palatine; naso palatine braches.etc.The mandibular nerve innervates the lower gum by its inferior alveolar lingual and buccal branches. Vessels in the gums usually accompany the nerves. Lymphatic of upper gum drain to the sub mandibular nodes and that of lower gum pass to the submental nodes and from its posterior part to the submandibular nodes.

Palate

The palate which forms the roof of the mouth has two distinct parts. The hard palate anteriorly and soft palate posteriorly.

Hard palate

Hard palate is the anterior portion of the floor of the mouth. It is formed by the maxillae and palatine bones. It is covered by mucous membrane. It forms a bony partition between the oral and nasal cavities. It also forms a rigid surface against which the tongue forces the food during chewing. The mucous on either side of raphe (a mid line ridge) is slightly corrugated, which helps to create friction. It is bounded in front and at the sides by the superior and inferior arches of alveolar process and gums and is continuous with soft palate posteriorly.

Soft palate

It is a mobile fold formed mostly of skeletal muscles. It forms the posterior portion of the roof of the mouth. It is an arch shaped muscular partition between oropharynx and naso pharynx and is lined by mucus membrane.

Hanging from free border of the soft palate is a conical muscular process called Uvula (grape). During swallowing the soft palate and the Uvula are drawn superiorly closing of the nasophrynx. This prevents swallowed food and liquids form entering the nasal cavity.

Tongue

The tongue together with associated muscle forms the floor of the oral cavity. It is composed of skeletal muscle covered with mucous membrane. The tongue is divided in to symmetrical lateral halves by a median septum that extend throughout its length and is attached inferiorly to the hyoid bone, styloid process of temporal bone and mandible.

The tongue has both intrinsic and extrinsic skeletal muscle fiber. The intrinsic muscles are confined with in the tongue and are not attached to the bone. Their muscle fibers which run in several different planes allow the tongue to change its shape becoming thicker, thinner, longer, or shorter, as needed for speech and swallowing. The extrinsic muscle extends to the tongue from their points of origin from the bones of the skull or the soft palate. These muscles help to alter its position. They protrude it, retract it, and move it from side to side.

The fold of mucosa called lingual phrenulum secures the tongue to the floor of the mouth. It also limits posterior movement of the tongue.

The superior tongue surface bears papillae, peg like projection of under lining mucosa. There are three types of papillae filiform, fungiform, and circumvillate.

The conical filiform papillae give the tongue surface a roughness that aids in licking semisolid foods (ice cream) and provide friction for manipulating food in the mouth. They contain keratin which stiffens them and gives the tongue its whitish appearance.

Fungiform papillae are mushroom like elevations distributed among the filiform papillae and are more numerous near the tip of the tongue. They appear as red dots on the surface of the tongue and most of them contain taste buds.

Circumlvillate are arranged in the form of an inverted v, in the posterior surface of the tongue and all of them contain taste buds. On the dorsum of the tongue are glands that secrete a digestive enzyme called lingual lipase which initiates digestion of triglycerides in to fatty acids and monoglycerides.

Teeth

The teeth (dentes) are accessory structures of digestive system located in sockets of alveolar process of the mandible and maxillae. The alveolar process is covered by the gums. The sockets are lined by peridental ligament which consists of dense fibrous connective tissue and is attached to socket walls and cementel surface of roof. It helps in anchoring the teeth in position and also acts as shock absorber during chewing.

A typical tooth consists of three principal regions. The crown is the visible portion above the level of gums. Embedded in the sockets or one to three roots. The neck is constricted junction line of crown and the root, near the gum line.

Teeth are composed of primarily of dentine, a calcified connective tissue layer that gives the tooth its basic shape and rigidity. Dentine encloses a cavity called pulp cavity which lies in the crown and filled with pulp.

Dentine of the crown is covered by layer of enamel which consists primarily of calcium phosphate and calcium carbonate. It is the hardest substance in the body. It protects tooth from wear of chewing and also acts as barrier against acids that could easily dissolve the dentin. Dentin of root is covered by cementum.

Dentition

Generally by the age of 21 two sets of teeth 1) primary (deciduous teeth-following off) or milk or baby teeth. 2) Permanent teeths are formed. Deciduoual teeth consists total number of 20 teeth they are 8 incisors, 4 canines, 8 molar teeth. Permanent teeth consists of total number of 32 teeth 8 incisors, 4 canines, 8 premolar, 12 molar teeth.

Salivary glands

A salivary gland is any cell or organ discharging secretion in to oral cavity. Saliva is a fluid that is continuously secreted in to mouth. Saliva 1) cleanses the mouth 2) dissolves food particle so that they can be tasted. 3) Moisten food and aids in compacting it in to bolos. 4) Contains enzyme that begin chemical breakdown of starchy food.

There are 3 pairs of salivary glands which lie outside the oral cavity and empty their secretion in to it they are parotid, submandibular, and sub lingual glands.

Parotid gland is largest gland lie anterior to ear, it runs parallel to the zygomatic arch pierces buccinatar muscle and opens in to vestibule, sub mandibular gland lies along the medial aspect of the mandibular body. It runs beneath the mucosa of oral cavity floor and opens at the base of the lingual frenulam. The small sublingual gland lies anterior to the submandibular gland under the tongue. It opens via 10 to 12 ducts in to the floor of the mouth.

Composition of saliva

Chemically saliva is 99.5% water and 0.5% solutes. Among the solutes are ions such as sodium, potassium, chloride, bicarbonate and phosphate. It also contains some dissolved gases and various organic substances including urea, uric acid serum albumin, globulin, mucus, bacterioliic enzyme (lisozome) and digestive enzyme (salivary amylase) which begins digestion of carbohydrates. Saliva is slightly acidic (pH 6.75 to 7) amount of saliva secreted daily varies considerably but average 1000- 1500 (70% by submandibular 25% by parotid and 5 % by sublingual glands)

Control of salivary glands

 Neural control Normally para sympathetic stimulation promotes continuous secretion of moderate amount of saliva. In contrast sympathetic stimulation dominates during stress resulting in dryness of mouth. Sympathetic stimulation constricts blood vessels and completely inhibits the salivary release.

Physiology of digestion in mouth

Mechanical digestion Through chewing or mastication the tongue manipulates food, the teeth grind it and the food is mixed with saliva. As result the food is mixed with saliva. As a result the food is reduced to a soft flexible mass called a bolus (lump) that is easily swallowed. Food molecules begin to dissolve in water in saliva an important activity because enzyme can only come into contact with food molecule in a medium.

Chemical digestion Two enzymes contribute to chemical digestion in the mouth salivary amylase and lingual lipase. Salivary amylase initiates the breakdown of starch. Lingual lipase secreted by glands in the tongue.

This enzyme starts the digestion of dietory fat in to fatty acids and monoglycerides.

Physiology of deglutition

The act of swallowing moves the food from the mouth to stomach. It is facilitated by saliva, mucous and involves the mouth, pharynx and oesophagus. Swallowing occurs in three stages.

1. Voluntary stage – in which bolus moves in to oropharynx.

2. The pharyngeal stage – involuntary passage of the bolus through the pharynx in to the   oesophagus

3. The esophageal stage – involuntary passage of bolus through the oesophagus in to the stomach.

Summary of functions of oral cavity

1. Analysis of material before swallowing
2. Mechanical pressing through the action of the teeth, tongue and palatal surface
3. Lubrication by mixing with mucous and salivary secretion
4. Limited digestion of carbohydrate and lipids

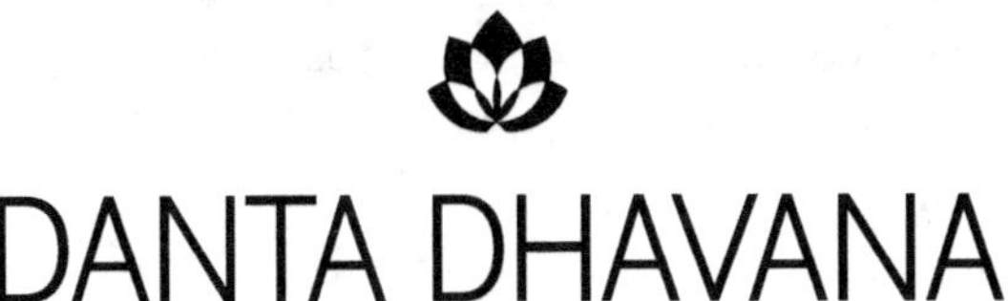

DANTA DHAVANA

Definition –

The process of the brushing and cleaning the teeth is called as *Danta Dhawana.*

Time-

Daily twice in the morning and before bedtime.

Material-

Ayurveda recommended medicinal plants that is pungent or astringent in taste and made up into soft brush. The fresh twigs of medicinal plants have property of Little fingers thickness and 12 fingers in length. When twigs are not available then the teeth should be cleaned with compound powder of medicinal plants. Karanja (Pongamia glabra), Karvira(Nerium Odorum), Malati(jasminum grandi florum), Arjuna (terminalia Arjuna), Vijaya Sara (terminalia Tomentosa), are used as fresh plant soft brush in Ayurveda. As Acharya sushruta is that nimba(Melia azadirachta), is the best fresh plant soft brush in in better rasa trees, Khadira(acacia katechu) best among kashaya rasa trees. Madhuka (basiya latifolia) is best among sweet Rasa trees and of the pungent trees karanja(Pongamia glabra) is the best.

Danta dhavna powder contents trikatu, trifala,Irimeda,Saindhava, Teja Patra etc. The Dantadhavana powder or paste slowly applied to top of teeth and gums.

Procedure

1.Use of medicinal plant fresh twig having *tikta, katu, kashaya rasa* eg. *Nimba, khadhira* also compound powder or paste should be used.

2.Fresh plant twigs are making like a brush structure and use gently without hurting gums

3.*Danta davana* powder or paste is rubbing on lower line of teeth then upper line with the help of little finger.

Benefits

- Remove the bad odour of the mouth
- Improve test and appetite
- It removes the dirt of tongue, teeth and mouth, thereby the taste for food is improved.

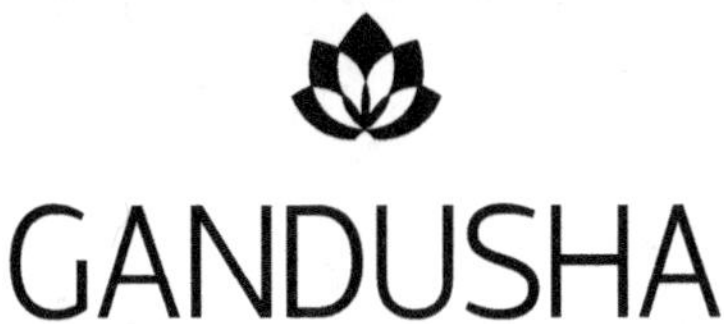

GANDUSHA

The word Gandusha is formed by Gadi + Gandescha which means mukha purnam i.e. filling the mouth.

Definition:

"*"Mukham asancharo yatu matra gandusha sa prakirtitaha"*"

Gandusha is the procedure of holding any liquid in the mouth to its full capacity without any movement inside. It is usually done with drava (liquid). One kola by measure is the dose of either a liquid or powder for gandusha.

Bheda[Types]

Based on doshagnata and karmukata Gandusha is classified mainly in to four. They are

- Snaihika (lubricating)   – indicated in diseases of vata
- Shamana (matigating)   – indicated in diseases of pitta
- Shodhana (purificatory)   - indicated in diseases of kapha
- Ropana (healing)   – indicated in ulcerations of mukha.

Synonyms for the above are shamana, stambhana, prasadana and nirvapana respectively.

Snaihika Gandusha

It is made from the dravyas, which are madhura, amla, lavana in rasa and ushna in veerya mixed with sneha dravyas and used warm. It is also made from mamsa rasa (meat soup), water or milk in which kalka of tila is mixed.

Shamana Gandusha

It is made from kashaya of dravyas which are madhura, tikta, kashaya in rasa and sheeta in virya such as patola, arishta, jambu, amra, madhuka, solution of sugar, madhu, dugdha, ikshu rasa, ghrita, etc.

Shodhana Gandusha

It is made from kashaya of dravyas that are katu, amla and lavana in rasa and ushna in virya and dravyas of shiro Virechana, sattu, madhya, mutra, and dhanyamla.

Ropana Gandusha

Dravyas used are having kashaya, madhura in rasa and shita ion virya or with such a dravyas mentioned in specific diseases.

Gandusha vidhi

The person is made to sit in a place devoid of heavy breeze but having sunlight, attentive towards treatment. He should be given mridu sweda and abhyanga over his gala, kapola, and lalata. He should be asked to hold the liquid in his mouth, raising his face little up. He should not drink the liquid. Filling the mouth with half, one third and one fourth of its capacity is the Pravara, Madhyama and avara matra respectively for liquid.

Again the person should be given mridhu sweda and abhyanga. Excited by these kapha moves into the mouth (from other parts). The liquid should be retained in the mouth till the cheeks show the signs of kapha accumulations and secretion of the ears in the nostrils and eyes or till the disappearance of the kapha by the action of the dravya.

In these way three, five, seven times gargles should be held or till the signs described under samyak dhoomapeeta lakshanas appear.

Age limitations -

Gandusha is contraindicated below the age of 5years.

Samyak Gandusha lakshana

-Swasthya (restoration of health)
  -Diminution of disorders
  -Filling of non sliminess (cleansing in the mouth)
  -Lightness of the mouth (freshness)
  -Clarity of sense organs (increased perception).

Heena yoga lakshana

-Appearance of jadhya (lassitude)
  -Arasa Jnana (loss of taste perception)
  -Aruchi (bad taste)
  -Praseka (excessive salivation)
  -Upalepa (coating of dirt inside the mouth)
  -Kaphothkesha (excitation of kapha)

Ati yoga lakshana

-Mukha Shosha (dryness of mouth)
  -Paka (Ulceration of oral cavity)
  -Klama (weakness)
  -Aruchi (loss of taste)
  -Hridaya drava (Discomfort in the chest region)
  -Svarasada (weakness of voice)
  -Karnanada (ringing in ears)
  -Trishna (thirst)

Gandusha dravas

Sneha, Ksheera, madhoodakam (honey water), saktu (fermented gravel), madhya, mamsa rasa, mutra (of animal), dhanyamla (wash of grains fermented by keeping over night)

Some daily usable gandusha dravas

- For daily use taila (tila) or mamsa rasa can be preferred.
- Water mixed with kalka of tila in danta shoola, danta chaala, and mukha rogas.
- Ksheera or ghrita can be used for osha, daha, paka, kshataja vrana and contact of visha, kshara, burns of fire.
- Madhu for removing sliminess, burning sensation, thirst and mukhapaka.
- Dhanyamla to remove asyavairasya, dirt and bad smell from the mouth.
- Sukhosna jala to get vaktra laghavata.

Gandusha anarha (contraindication)

Persons suffering from visha, Moorcha, mada, Shosha, Raktapitta, kupita akshi mala, ksheena and ruksha rogi.

Gandush in Dinacharya

Kashaya of ksheri vriksha has to be used for washing the mukha for Swastha person to prevent diseases that may be caused due to rakta and pitta.

Dalhana commenting on this opines that ksheerivriksha means nyagrodhadi gana dravyas. Kashaya of this is used for gandush (antarmukha prakshalana) to prevent or cure rakta dusthi janya vyadhis.

Kwatha of ksheeri vriksha is used for kavalagraha to alleviate arochaka, asyavairasya, malinata, pooti (mukha dourgandata) and praseka.

Gandusha in dinacharya has been explained with to intentions (objectives).

1) Preventive (prevention of the diseases)

2) Helth promotive (by improving the oral hygiene)

Tila taila has been mentioned for nitya gandusha and benefits are explained as fallows. It gives strength to hanu sandhi, improves voice, does proper upachaya (nourishment) of vadana (oral mucosa), and improves taste perception. Person will not suffer from Kantha Shosha, cracking of the lips, no falling of teeth. Gum tissue becomes firm. There will be no danta harsha or danta shoola.

General mode of action of Gandusha

Even though gandusha is sthanika chikitsa its action can be understood as both

> 1) Local action
> 2) Systemic action

1) Local action:

Gandusha has many actions locally they are as follows
- Increases local defense mechanism.
- Enhancing both mechanical and chemical digestion of food that starts in the mouth.
- Removing of metabolic wastes (urea and uric acid),
- Soothing effect.
- Strengthening of muscles of oral cavity.

The action of gandusha (holding mouthful of liquid) exerts increased mechanical pressure inside the oral cavity. So this increased pressure stimulates pressoreceptor (stretch reflex) that are present in the mouth. Once the pressoreceptor is stimulated they send signals to salivary nuclei in the brain stem (pons and medulla). As a result Para sympathetic nervous system activity increases and motor fibres in facial (VII) and glossopharyngial (IX) nerve trigger dramatically increased out put of saliva. Chemical constituent present in the drug also stimulate chemoreceptors present in the mouth, which in turn increases salivary secretions. An enzyme called lysosome present in saliva is bacteriostatic in action .It will not allow for the growth of pathogenic microorganisms in the oral cavity. Antibody IgA present in saliva also provide protection against microorganisms. Thus gandusha increases local defense mechanism.

The enzyme salivary amylase present in saliva ands lingual lipase secreted by the lingual gland present at the dorsum of the tongue initiates digestion of carbohydrate and fats respectively. Gandusha increases secretions of these enzymes.

Excessive salivary secretion, which predominantly contains water, removes metabolic wastes present in oral cavity.

Some of dravyas used for gandusha like panchavalkala produces soothing effect on lesions like ulcers thus prevents ulcers from physical and chemical injury.

The act of gandusha and kavala gives proper exercise to the muscles of cheeks, tongue, lips and soft palate there by increasing the motor functions of these muscles.

2] Systemic action

Mucosal layer inferior to the tongue (sublingual) is thin and highly vascular enough to permit the rapid absorption of the lipid soluble drugs into systemic circulation. Some of the drugs irritates the oral mucosa (by their chemical nature) and increases vascular permeability. Thus an active principle of dravya gets absorption in systemic circulation. Most of the dravas (kwatha) given for gandusha are warm (sukhoshna) so raised temperature causes the increased vascular permeability there by enhancing systemic absorption of drugs.

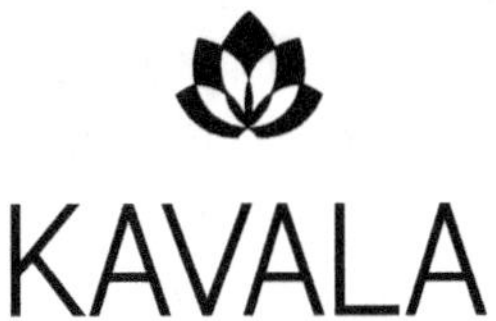

CHAPTER SIX

KAVALA

The quantity which can be easily and conveniently rolled out in the mouth is the proper dose in respect of a *Kavala*, where as one which can not be so easily and conveniently rolled out in the mouth is called as *Gandusha*.

Kavala is a variety of the gargling. It is important to Gargle the mouth after meals, eating any food and after brushing the teeth. One should use cold or lukewarm water, Tila tail or cold milk for gargling. Gargling with lukewarm water exerts cleaning action on the mouth, teeth, gums and tongue. It imparts a light and fresh feeling to the mouth. Gargling with oil exerts a cleansing and strengthening action on tongue, teeth, mouth and voice.

Kavala can be defined as holding medicated semisolids or liquids in the mouth in such a quantity so that it could be rolled out in the mouth.

In *Gandusha*, the fluid penetrates the oral mucosa and gums and exerts its specific action. In *Kavala*, it exerts a soothing and cleansing action on the mouth. In *Dincharya*, mainly *Kavala Upkrama* is advised.

TYPES OF KAVALA:

Gandusha and *Kavala* are both variants of gargling. *Gandusha* and *Kavala* are of four different types: *Kavala* may be divided into four kind's i. e. *Snehika, Shamana, Shodhan* and *Ropan*.

Gandusha is of four kinds viz. *snaihika*(oleating), *shamana*(palliative), *shodhan*(purifactory) and *ropana*(healing), likewise is *Kavala*.

Snaihika is done in disease of *vata* with drugs possessing *snigdha* and *ushna* properties, in diseases of *pitta* with drugs possessing *swadu* and *shita*, for *kapha* shodhan with drugs possesing *katu,amla,lavana* and *ushna*; for healing of ulcers with drugs possessing *kashay,tikta* and *madhura* are used.

1) *Snehika Kavala:*

Til kalka, water, milk and sneha are useful for the vataj diseases of the mouth i. e. diseases associated with dryness and roughness in the mouth.

2) *Shaman or Prasadana Kavala:*

Milk and sugar medicated with sweet and old medicines is used for its soothing action on Pittaj diseases of the mouth. e.g. stomatitis or ulcers in the mouth and gums.

3) *Shodhan Kavala:*

Decoction of medicines with astringent, sour or salty taste is used for its cleansing action in *Kaphaj* diseases of the mouth, characterized by excessive salivation and stickiness in the mouth.

4) *Ropan Kavala:*

The healing gargles should be composed of bitter, astringent, sweet, pungent, heat making articles and should be employed in cases of ulceration of the mouth.

PROCEDURE OF KAVALA:

The person should sit in a place devoid of breeze. The neck, cheeks and the forehead of the patient to be treated with *Kavala* should be massaged and fomented. The patient during the use of a *Kavala*, should sit in an erect posture, keeping his face slightly lifted up and in the least distracted state.

A material which is to be gargled should be hold in mouth and then should gargled properly and should be spit out; the whole procedure should be repeated for three to four minutes. He should continue to do *Kavala* till eyes and nose start watering.

An amelioration of the disease, a sense of lightness and purity in the mouth, a cheerful fame of mind and an exhilarating vigor in the organs of sense are the features which mark an act of prefect and satisfactory *Kavala*.

A sense of physical lassitude, salivation and a defect in the sense of fatigue and inflammation of the mouth are the symptoms of *asamyak Kavala*.

ADVANTAGES AND IMPORTANCE OF KAVALA:

Diseases of the neck, head, ear, mouth and eyes; excess salivation, disease of the throat, dryness of the mouth, nausea, stupor, anorexia and rhinitis are curable especially by Kavala.

In conditions like *Dantachal* of the teeth, shaky teeth and diseases of the mouth like *mukhapaka* and *mukhavrana*, *Kavala* of water mixed with paste of tila, either lukewarm or cold, is good or daily use with either oil or soup of meat i.e. *mansa rasa* for gargles. Keeping of oil, milk, ghee gargles provides strength in jaws and voice, development of face, maximum taste and relish in food. The person does not suffer from dryness of throat, there is no fear of lip cracking, teeth are not affected by caries; rather they become firm rooted. Teeth become able to chew even the hardest food.

CONTRAINDICATION FOR KAVALA:

Kavala is contraindicated in unconscious, poisoned, weak or marasmic persons or persons suffering from bleeding disorders and conjunctivitis.

Gandusha and Kavala Difference:

Both these are explained as *bahya roopi shaman chikitsa* in most of *urdhvajatrugata vikaras* especially *mukha roga. Gandusha* differs from *kavala* in following aspects.

1) Quantity of *Dravya* - Quantiy of *dravya* that is to be retained in mouth in *gandusha* is to its full capacity. Where as in *kavala* quantity is such that *dravya* can be moved inside the mouth.

2) Movement of *Dravya* - in gandusha *dravya* that is retained in mouth should not be moved. In *kavala drava* can be moved inside.

3) *Vaya* or *Avastha anusasra*—in childhood and old age usually *kavala* is preferred. Because in children proper tone of the muscles of oral cavity is not attained so to strengthen it act of *kavala* is to be performed. In old age muscles becomes flaccid and loose their tonicity due to degenerative changes. Hence *kavala* is indicated.

4) *Dravya swaroopa* (consistency)—the *swaroopa* of *dravya* in *kavala* is usually *kalka* where as in case of *gandusha* it is *drava*.

5) Indication in *vyadhis*---usually *gandusha* is preferred in condition of oral cavity characterized by *vedana, shotha, srava* as *drava* is not moved inside the mouth otherwise it aggravates condition. *Kavala* is indicated in the *vyadhis* where there is more *kapha sanchaya* in mouth, *guruta, jadhya, alasya (kaphaja Vyadhi), ardita*.

But generally indication, *samyak, heena, atiyog lakshanas* and benefits of both *kavala and gandusha* are considered to be same.

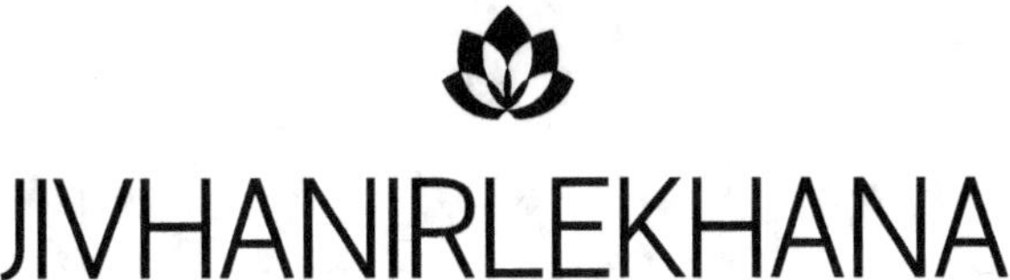

CHAPTER SEVEN

JIVHANIRLEKHANA

Definition

The process of cleaning the tongue by using tongue cleaner of gold, silver or copper is called as *Jivhanirlekhana.*

Time

After the dental procedure.

Material

Jivhanirlekhana done with the help of the smooth and flexible file of gold, silver or copper. Even of medicinal plant tricks itself which should be 10 fingers in the length

Procedure

Gently rubbed tongue paper the tongue after dental procedure.

Benefits

1. It gives relief and removes the bad taste.
    2. It removes the bad odour of the month.

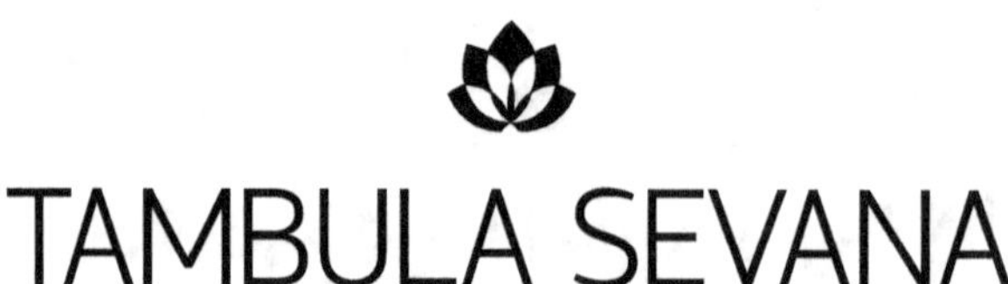

CHAPTER EIGHT

TAMBULA SEVANA

Ayurvedic classics mentioned tambula sevana in the context of Dinacharya for the maintenance of perfect oral hygiene and as a preventive modality to avoid diseases of the oral cavity. In the present situation, many people are habituated to paan chewing along with harmful substances like tobacco, which has given rise to several problems like bleeding gums, bad odor of mouth and breath, mouth ulcers, adverse dental conditions and dreadful disorders like cancer of the oral cavity. Tambula has positive effects on health if taken in an appropriate way as explained in our classics. Different concepts related to tambula sevana are relevant even for the current lifestyle, where primary prevention comes into action.

Drugs used for Tambul preparation:

Jatiphal – Jayphal (Myristica fragrans)
   Latakasturi - Abelmoschus moschatus (Muskadana)
   Pugphala (*supari*) - areca-nut
   Lavanga - clove
   Kankol- piper cubela
   Tambul patra – Leaf of *Nagarvel* plant (Beetle leaf)
   Karpura- Cinnamomum camphora
   Ela – cardamomum

Procedure:

Available drugs mentioned for *Tambula* preparation taking in proportion rolled in Beetle leave for chewing and holding.

Benefits:

1.Cleaning of oral cavity.
   2.Develops taste and mouth freshening.

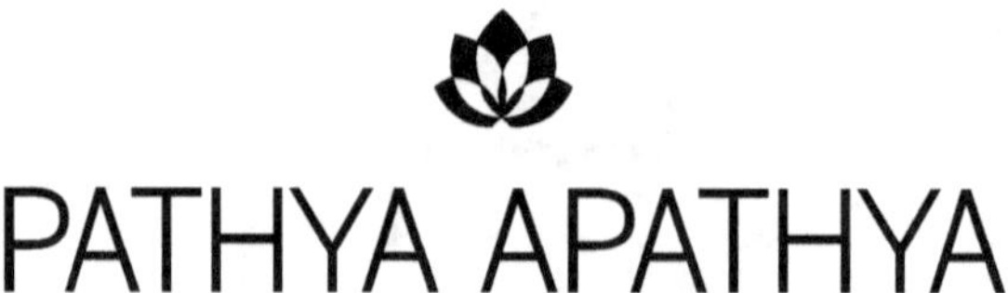

CHAPTER NINE

PATHYA APATHYA

PATHYA:

Acceptable diet and acceptables regimens for oral health are listed below:

- *Mudga yusha - Dal* pepared with Moong
- Meat soup
- *Katu* and Bitter rasa juices
- Gargles of *Haridra* and Alum mixture
- Decoction of *Khadira,ghritam,katu* and bitter rasa juices
- Fruits-Awala, Orange, Papaya, Apple etc.
- Green vegetables
- Daily routines -*Danta Dhavana,Gandusha, Kavala,Jivhanirlekhana* etc.
- Ayurved drugs- Musali, shatavari, Karvellaka, Leaves of Patola, Raw radish, Karpurambu, Betel leaves

APATHYA :

- One should not keeping his face downwards durring sleep
- One should not sleep durring day time
- Edibles that are difficult to chew and digest
- Virudha Aahara e.g. fish + milk

- Eating of curd durring dinner time
- Excessive eating of sweet diet e.g. Jaggery

Bibliography

1. Sushruta Samhita with Nibandha Sangraha commentary - Yadavaji Trikamaji Acharya.
2. Astanga Hridaya with Sarvanga sundara commentary of Arunadatta and of Hemadri - P.V. Sharma.
3. Charaka Samhita with Ayurveda Deepika commentary by Chakrapani - Yadavaji Trikamaji
4. AcharyAstanga Samgraha with Shashilekha commentary of Indu - Panditrao and Vaidya Ayodhya pandeya.
5. Bhavaprakasha with Vidyotini Hindi commentary - Brahmashankar Mishra.
6. Sharangadhara Samhita with Adhamalla's Deepika and Kashiram's Goodhartha Deepika commentary - Pandit Parashuram Shastri Vidyasagara Varanasi.
7. Yogaratnakara by Indra Deva Tripati and Dayashankar Tripathi.1st editionPublished by Krishnadas academy
8. Yogaratnakara with Vidyotini Hindi commentary by Vaidya Lakshmipathi Shastri - Bhishagratna Brahmashankar Shastri.
9. Madhava Nidana with Madhukosha commentary by Vijayaraksita and Srikantadatta published b Published by Choukumbha Sanskrit Bhavana
10. Bhaishajya Ratnavali with Vidyotini Hindi vyakhya, vimarsha parishishta sahita byAmbikadatta Shastri. Published by Choukumbha Sanskrit Bhavana.14st edition.
11. Amara Kosha Satippana maniprabha, Hindi teekopeta by Hargovind Shastri.5th edition Published by Choukumbha Sanskrit Bhavana
12. Ayurvedic pharmacology and therapeutic uses of medicinal plants - Vaidya Vishnumahadev Gogte.
13. Shabda kalpa Druma – Vol-III,
14. Abhinava Shareera prathama bhaga ,by Damodar sharma gouda.1st edition 1974.published by Baidynath Ayurveda bhavana Pvt Ltd.
15. Agni Puranaki Ayurvediya anusandhanatmaka sameeksha.published by Shri Satguru Publication. 1st edition 2000
16. Text Book of Bhaishajya Kalpana by Shobha Hirematha. Published by T.B.M Prakashana, 1st edition 2000

17. Bhaishajya Kalpana Vijnana, by Ram Chandra reddy. Published by Choukumbha Sanskrit Bhavana.1ˢᵗ edition 1998.

18. Gray's Anatomy - peter C.Williams, 37ᵗʰedition 1992.

19. Principles of Anatomy and Physiology by G.J Tortora and S.R.Grabowski, Harper Collins college publishers, 8ᵗʰedition 1996.

20. Human Anatomy and Physiology by Elaine Marieb R.N PhD Benjamin/ Cummings science publishing. 4ᵗʰedition.

21. Diseases of E.N.T by P.L. Dingra, published by Elsevier, a division Reed Elsevier India pvt ltd.3ʳᵈedition.

22. Text Book of of E.N.T by Mohd.Maqbool.published by Jaypee brothers Medical Publishers Pvt.Ltd. 6ᵗʰedition

23. Mukhswastham by Dr Vipul Patit, 1ˢᵗ edition,2019 chapter 1ˢᵗ.